STICK-TO-IT-IVENESS

STICK-TO-IT-IVENESS

Lessons Learned from Drums, Dogs, & Sports

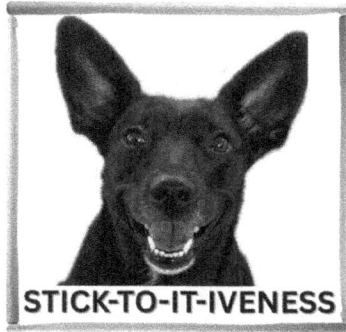

Jacob Morris

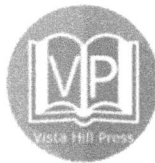

Vista Hill Press

A Division of Five Minute Network, LLC

Los Angeles

STCIK-TO-ITIVENESS:
Lessons Learned from Drums, Dogs, & Sports

Copyright © 2025 by Jacob Morris

Published by
Vista Hill Press
A Division of Five Minute Network, LLC
907 Westwood Blvd., Suite 405
Los Angeles, CA 90024

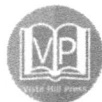

First Edition: 2025
Production & Marketing Manager: Jacob Morris
Logo design: Jacob Morris
Cover design: Bojan Rekovic
Book design: Julia Bleck
Library of Congress Cataloging-in-Publication Data is available
ISBN-13: 978-0-9968377-8-1
ISBN-13: 978-0-9968377-9-8

For Mom and Dad—for "sticking" with me even when it wasn't easy.

For my Papa and my Gramma—for teaching me the most important values and setting me up for the future.

For our dogs Zoey and Luca—for always being adorable and being there for me. And to our late dog Benny--for being a bundle of love.

CONTENTS

Introduction 1

Discipline 9

Initiative 15

Courage 19

Perseverance 29

Forgiveness 37

Patience 43

Healthy Lifestyle 47

Values Into Action 53

Hobbies 61

Family 69

Community 77

Collaboration 93

Listening 107

Conclusion 111

Acknowledgements 115

Information About The Author 119

INTRODUCTION

The major loves of my life are my dogs, Camp Kesem, sports, videography and playing the drums. Yeah, I am passionate about a lot of things. Though the connection between these five very different entities is not immediately obvious, my passions actually have a lot in common in terms of the life lessons they have taught me. These lessons have changed my life for the better and I'm hoping they might be helpful to you as well.

To understand where I started, I think it's helpful to share a bit about my early life. My story begins with repeated ear infections which began shortly after birth. When I turned one, my ear doctor discovered the reason I wasn't walking, talking, or even babbling was that I couldn't hear anything. It was as though I had spent the first year of my life living underwater. My parents tell me I stood up and walked for the first time three days after having tubes placed to drain the water from my ears which restored my hearing. Even though I could finally hear sounds, it took time to catch up and understand the concept of speech and how sounds could be used to communicate. It took much of my childhood to fully resolve my hearing problems but thankfully, my hearing is now completely normal.

I don't remember much of my life before my mom got cancer. The spring I turned six was already more than full of excitement and changing times for me. Literally in the span of one month, I experienced my first evacuation due to wildfires, had to postpone my eagerly awaited 6th birthday party due to bad air quality, and my family moved into a new house just a week before my preschool graduation. I looked to my parents to guide me through all these events and milestones and trusted that no matter what I faced, I would be all right as long as I had their love and support. My dad had a long commute and worked long hours, so my mom was the constant presence in my and my three sisters' lives, so she was the one who took care of our day-to-day needs. My mom pretty much ensured our busy family was organized and got everything done.

I realized everything was about to change when my parents called me and my three sisters into the family room, sat us down on the couch, and told us the terrifying news. Even at an incredibly young age, I understood what my parents were telling us. My mom had cancer.

I was distraught by the news and didn't want to believe it was true. I didn't have time to process what was happening because suddenly, my mom had what seemed like constant doctor's appointments and tests and my dad was suddenly the one driving us places and taking care of things at home. Even my preschool graduation ceremony was affected as my mom got an emergency call to go to an unexpectedly available appointment with her surgeon and my dad was the one who stayed with my sisters to watch my ceremony. Then, instead of my highly anticipated graduation dinner, he drove all of us to join my mom at the hospital to learn the treatment plan for her cancer.

My mom immediately began treatments for her cancer which included chemotherapy, which caused her beautiful hair to fall out. Even with her terrible situation and while she was still in active treatment, my mom still thought about her children and found the summer camp that would become a huge part of my life.

My early challenges with hearing and speech and growing up with a mom with cancer were certainly difficult. However, they laid the groundwork for many of the strengths I later developed. I'll tell you more as in the pages that follow. I've learned that challenges can sometimes be the most important means for us to grow and become stronger. For example, the challenges I have faced and overcome in my life inspired me to write this book to share my journey. Dealing with a speech delay and hearing loss from a very young age combined with my mom's cancer diagnosis resulted in me being a kid who was initially afraid of taking risks. New situations such as public speaking used to be very difficult for me. However, new situations no longer scare me. I've learned to embrace new situations and see them as opportunities for growth. I guess challenges can slow us down or they can strengthen us and build up our creative and confidence muscles. I know they did for me and I'm hoping they can do the same for you because we all face challenges in life. None of us are immune to that. How we deal with these challenges is our choice and that choice determines our future.

I am so grateful for the support and encouragement from my parents who have always been in my corner. As I reach the end of my childhood and begin to turn the corner to adult life, I now realize that my parents helped me maneuver the roadblocks of life and help me gain the values and life skills that I needed so that I could mature into a kind, hard-working, collaborative member of my community.

I know I'm biased here but I have to say that having dogs in my life has also been a hugely important factor in my development as a person. I believe that dogs can be critically important to family life. You can call yourself a family without a dog, and many people do, but there is nothing like having a dog to bring a family together. Just as I think a dog is important for family life, I also think pursuing your passions is necessary for a person to live a truly satisfying life. Aside from my dogs, my passions are sports, playing the drums, and Camp Kesem. You are probably wondering what Camp Kesem is. Don't worry, I'll tell you all about Camp Kesem and all your questions will be answered about this life-changing camp and charity! Trust me, you will likely be inspired just reading about the impact of this amazing organization.

I hope you find my story helpful. It is my goal to help other kids and young adults realize that they are not alone and that there are steps you can take to build your confidence and life skills. I am sharing what worked for me, but each person is different. The important thing is to find the activities that you love doing and support you, your family, and your community. Usually these are the activities that you do on your own when no one is making you do them. These are the activities that help you grow as a person, and your growth will positively affect those around you. The only caveat I'll add before getting started is that I think everyone should have a dog if possible. There is no substitute for having the unconditional love of a dog, especially a rescue dog.

DISCIPLINE

To me, it all starts with discipline. Discipline means doing the right thing even when no one is watching. This means ensuring that you act in ways that are in keeping with your goals for yourself and your values. Of course, to develop discipline, it's essential to be consistent with your behavior and habits on a moment by moment basis. Many people associate discipline as something generally learned through schoolwork and the academic world. For me, I have learned discipline through playing the drums, having dogs, and playing sports.

To start off with, let me describe how I came to love the drums. Once I started playing the drums in fourth grade, it quickly became apparent that the only way to progress in my musical skills was to have the discipline to practice every day. Some days, it was easy. I wanted to play the drums on those days so playing came naturally. Other days were a different story. On those days, I didn't want to play. However, the key for me was to play even when I didn't want to play.

Taking care of dogs was much the same. Taking care of another living being means doing the right things whether you feel like it or not. After years of begging for a dog, I was thrilled when my parents finally agreed to adopt our dog Benny from a local rescue shelter when I was nine. Benny was a King Charles Cavalier-Maltese mix with a lot of personality and a lot of strong opinions. As most children do when they want a dog, I promised to do my part to help feed, walk, and clean up after our new dog. Once we got Benny, I quickly learned that dogs thrive on routine and that requires those who take care of them to have the discipline to ensure a defined schedule. Dogs rely on us for everything. A happy dog learns to follow rules when we establish consistency in feeding, training and walking; without this, you will have an out-of-control, untrainable dog (and likely one who will make the house their bathroom). To keep your dog healthy and happy, and to be able to enjoy their companionship, consistency is key. This takes discipline. The responsibility of taking care of dogs since such an early age has certainly allowed me to improve this skill. This has helped me to become more conscientious about doing my jobs in my everyday life. Very few kids feel like doing homework when there are so many more fun things you could be doing. Through the discipline I learned from the act of walking my dog every day, I developed the internal strength to make myself do my homework every day.

Having to wake up early and walk the dogs every day taught me how to consistently do hard tasks even when I really would prefer to not do them. I remember many early mornings when Benny scratched at my bedroom door begging me to take him for a walk. I loved Benny and wanted to show my parents I could keep my word, so I learned to wake up early and walk Benny on his preferred route through our neighborhood which took twenty minutes. This meant I had to get up earlier than usual for Benny to take care of him each morning before school. It didn't matter if it was cold and rainy or hot and miserable outside; you have to walk your dog every day. In this case, my mom was very busy in the mornings, and she sometimes didn't feel well due to chemotherapy. Benny had a lot of energy and needed his morning walk every day so he wouldn't be bouncing off the walls while my sisters and I were in school. At the end of each walk, Benny would be panting, but the second he got inside, he was ready to play again. Benny had too much energy and love to share. This meant there was no time for rest with dogs and no days off. Having a dog is a full-time commitment which certainly teaches discipline if you're willing to learn. That willingness is a big key.

Another key is showing the skills of leadership. With dogs, you either set the tone with them, or they will set the tone with you. I learned it was important to become a leader for the dogs so they could learn the skills they needed. When we got Benny, he was 3 years old, and he did not listen much to us. He was a rescue and had been through a lot and it was difficult for him to listen with all the anxiety he had. Over time, with a lot of love and leadership from us, Benny learned to relax and listen and that meant more "Benny love" for all of us.

INITIATIVE

Once you've developed your skills with discipline, the next skill to work on is initiative. Discipline is doing the right thing even when no one is watching you. Initiative is the energy needed to do the right things. It's the energy to solve problems. It's the energy to listen. It's the energy to improve yourself and your community. These skills are certainly intertwined. Our dog Benny was abandoned to a shelter when he was three years old. After that, two other families adopted him and returned him to the shelter. Knowing that makes it easy to understand why Benny was so anxious and scared much of the time. When we met Benny at the shelter, I noticed that Benny showed initiative when he ran over and licked my sister's foot to get her attention. Benny didn't wait for us to notice him. He took the initiative to show his loving and adorable side, and we were so blessed to have the opportunity to welcome him into our family.

Initiative requires focus as paying attention is critical to whatever task you're doing. With dogs, you can't take your eyes off them for too long or else they can get themselves into trouble. I remember when one of our other dogs, Zoey, was a puppy and she got hold of a battery and she bit into it. We had to rush her to the veterinarian and fortunately she was ok. The veterinarian told us that it could have been very serious if we hadn't stopped Zoey from swallowing the battery. She only ended up with a cracked tooth. Luckily, we got Zoey medical attention in time, and she didn't have any long term problems from the battery acid, but this taught me a lot about focus and initiative to help keep our loved ones safe. After Zoey's accident, I became more focused with Benny and I noticed that he would pick up woodchips, plastic, and other small objects in his mouth. We always reacted quickly and removed the objects from his mouth before he could swallow them. Without focus and initiative, Benny could have been seriously hurt.

COURAGE

So far, we've talked about having the discipline to do the right things even when no one is watching, and we've talked about having the initiative to do so. Now I'd like to mention what supplies the strength to have discipline and initiative; that's courage. Yes, the courage from The Wizard of Oz. It takes courage to do the right things. It's not easy. In life, many situations are scary and difficult to maneuver. Life isn't easy. Sometimes we prefer to play it safe and not risk much. However, doing so too often can lead to stagnation and prevent growth. It isn't good to never challenge yourself or put yourself in uncomfortable situations. As is the case with most things in life, the perfect mix of risk is somewhere in the middle. The key is to take some calculated risks some of the time and this takes courage. In my life, I have taken a lot of risks, most at the time I really was scared to do so. Whether it be drums, switching schools, or playing sports, there were plenty of times when I felt scared and I had to summon a lot of courage.

One example of me taking risks comes from the drums. My favorite part of playing the drums is when all of the parts of the drum set are tuned to perfection and the sound that comes out is just unlike anything you have ever heard. I also love leading the band into songs, controlling the tempo, and responding to the music that they play. Even when I mess up, (which happens to everyone eventually), I always love to get back on track and continue playing. I don't love it when I mess up, as I want to play my parts as well as possible every time, but that will never happen, no matter how much anyone practices. Everyone is human, and humans are not perfect.

After I began playing the drums, I decided I wanted to attend a music camp to improve my skills. When I first arrived, I felt really nervous. I felt like I was outmatched, even though looking back on it, no one there was any more experienced at their respective instruments than I was. As a little kid, I felt like I didn't belong. I got assigned to my respective group and started practicing and learning. Over the next two weeks, my group and I practiced many songs until we performed them all. I remember feeling nervous on the day of the performance, but I played all my songs well and felt great about how things went. Like I have said before, performing with a group is an amazing feeling. Over the next few years, I attended this camp, eventually getting moved up to a higher skill level group.

Eventually, I started to work at the camp as a counsellor, and I became even more skilled at the drums. I can credit this camp and the people who helped me there with developing my musical skills and also my skills in working with others. Looking back now, I see that I couldn't have done this without courage.

Changing schools is always a difficult situation. Doing it multiple times is even more difficult. That is what I have had to do throughout my childhood. Due to numerous of events beyond my control, I have had to switch schools. Whether it be due to my family moving, the amount of violence at a school, or a myriad of other reasons, changing schools became a necessity. The switch from school to school is very difficult. For academic reasons, it is very challenging as you have to learn in an entirely new environment with brand new teachers and sometimes a new curriculum. It is also challenging as you have to make new friends. Despite this, I have persevered and have had a good amount of success adjusting to new situations throughout my many years attending school. I have achieved this success by continuing to do what I love, no matter where I find myself; and much of this is through music.

I have always loved to play music, so I have always found myself with the musical crowd at whatever school I attend. It can be a school orchestra, small bands that play popular music, or another type of musical group. I found ways to find the people with whom I most connect who are often the musicians. I share a creative spirit with them and that helps form bonds of friendship and collaboration. By spending time with them, I have been able to build relationships with like-minded individuals. This strategy can be used by anyone even if you're not a musician. Try to find a group of people who truly understands you and with whom you can truly be yourself. For me, it is musicians, but for someone else, it could be sports fans, history buffs, or any other hobby or interest. Being able to play the drums at any school I attended greatly benefited my ability to find ways of enjoying school and making friends, even when things seemed challenging. The people I have met through playing the drums at school have helped me form friendships with a great group of people

When I first met my drum instructor, who I called "Mr. Larry," I felt a bit nervous. He was an older, tall, bald guy who I didn't think was going to be very kind when I first met him. However, as I got to know him, I realized that he was actually really nice and supportive. During our first lesson, he was incredibly patient with me and so I was eager to return to improve my drumming skills. Every time I returned to take a lesson, he was willing to help me with whatever music I needed help. Whether it be music that I had to learn for school or just any song that I liked at the time, he would help me learn how to play it.

I remember one time I suggested a very complex song that I wanted to learn, and I spent the entire lesson with him explaining the small details in the song. I remember the incredible feeling when I finally could play the song near the end of the lesson. This was how most of the lessons we had would go. At a different time, my sister suggested a song for me to learn so I took it to Mr. Larry and asked him to help me learn it. However, he was stumped by the song. This showed me that he was human and wasn't able to play every song ever created without breaking a sweat. The next lesson we had, we finally figured out the song and the feeling of accomplishment was wonderful. Sometimes he would help me with a piano part for a song. Sometimes he would help me with a snare drum part. Sometimes he would help me with another element to the song. I started to look forward to this process and the struggle to figure out the music became a sort of puzzle that was so much fun to figure out.

Whenever I couldn't figure out a song, I made sure to go home and practice it a ton so I could easily play the song for the next lesson. I remember one time; he invited me to go to a concert he was performing at a local restaurant. When I got there, I saw him sitting on the drum set, playing away. It was wonderful to see him so locked into the performance that he did not even notice me in the crowd. I imagined how much courage he must have needed over the years to get to that level.

Another time when I needed courage from my time playing sports in high school. In high school, I decided to start playing baseball again. I hadn't played organized baseball since elementary school, but I love the sport and wanted to try it again. When I got back onto the field, I felt completely outmatched. I hadn't swung at a pitch in years and during that time my swing wasn't what it used to be. Some would never have put themselves back in that situation, but I really wanted to play baseball again and play on the school team. After a year of riding the bench and practicing to show my coaches how much better I had become, I finally got my chance to start at second base. The first time I walked into the batter's box, I was terrified, and the pitcher looked so intimidating. As the pitcher started to throw the first pitch, I gripped the bat extremely tight and watched a pitch go right past me for strike one. The notion of swinging did not even come across my mind. I was afraid of embarrassing myself in front of the crowd. I told myself to give it a shot and swing and hope for the best. The pitcher began to throw the next pitch and my muscles tensed and I just couldn't bring the bat down from my shoulder as strike two whizzed right past me. I stepped out of the batter's box and called for time from the umpire. My heart was pounding. I had finally gotten my chance to play on the team after all the hard work I had put in, and all I could think about was not making myself look like a fool. I took a deep breath and stepped back into the batter's box. I stared the pitcher and got myself ready to swing and swing I did. I swung incredibly hard, but just like in the short story "Casey At The Bat," I missed, and the ball hit the catcher's mitt, and the umpire signaled that I was out. I walked back to the dugout. Some may have been sad that they got out so quickly and easily, but I saw it differently. I may not have made contact with the pitch, but I did not go down looking. I hadn't swung a baseball bat in a live game for years, yet I still tried, and at the end of the day, that is all you can do in life. You can only try your best to success. Sometimes you succeed and sometimes you fail. However, if you never try, you will never succeed. A few months after that game, I was still on the team, and I had gotten lots of hits. My confidence was soaring. I would never have gotten to that level if I hadn't swung at the pitch even though I was scared to swing the bat, fearing embarrassing myself. Without courage, I would never have gotten a single hit ever, let alone thrive at the plate.

PERSEVERANCE

Unfortunately, life always includes hardships and tragedies. I know that I have experienced a few in my life. However, you can't let these control your life. I'm not saying you can't be frustrated or mourn a loss, but don't let it control you. If you do, you will find yourself throwing away precious time. This is about perseverance, which is about continuing even when things get difficult.

When we got our second dog Zoey, Benny became very jealous and did not seem to like her. However, as time went on, Zoey would follow Benny around and just try to be his friend. I noticed that Benny started to bond with her more. They would start to play, and Zoey looked up to him like a big brother. It was difficult for Zoey when Benny died. I'm not sure what Zoey understood, but she seemed to become very sad until we got our third dog Luca who instantly bonded with her.

The importance of perseverance was brought home to me by seeing how Zoey dealt with Benny's death. When Benny died, Zoey became heartbroken and depressed.

Benny was family for her so it was a major loss for her. Zoey had less energy, less "drive", and was not herself after Benny passed. No matter how much we showed her love, she struggled to be herself after the loss of Benny. My family and I had an idea. Some people have emotional support dogs, but at this time, Zoey herself needed an emotional support dog. We looked and looked and eventually came across a rescue dog, who we named Luca. We got Luca from a rescue who takes dogs from South Korea and brings them to safety in America. When we first were introduced to Luca, we were told he was extremely scared. She was extremely afraid likely because of what he had experienced before he was saved. Zoey instantly looked better as soon as she met Luca. Moreover, Zoey became the "Benny" of Luca's life, and Luca started to improve. Zoey finally had a dog to interact with after the passing of her brother, and she instantly bonded with Luca. I remember how she patiently waited at the stairs and showed Luca that they weren't scary. She stood on the stairs until Luca was brave enough to follow her upstairs. Zoey showed how, even after a tragedy of losing someone she loved, she was still able to show another dog love. Luca desperately needed love as well after a scary start to his life.

This is all about perseverance and moving forward with love.

Zoey would teach Luca a lot of things when we first got him. Zoey and Luca would play, which Zoey always wanted to do with Benny, even when he was not physically able to do so. Luca was very young and was able to play with Zoey, which she enjoyed a ton. A few years later now, Luca and Zoey still love each other just as much as they did when they first met. Luca has grown in size to be around the same size as Zoey.

All the love that Zoey has shown Luca has helped him move on from his rocky start to his life. Now, he is extremely loving, confident, and happy. I am not sure if Luca would have grown to be this functioning without the unconditional love that he received from Zoey, along with the love that he received from our family. I still believe Zoey remembers and misses Benny, as she truly did love him. I think that she sees a little bit of Benny in Luca which is why she instantly loved him so much. They actually look a bit alike. I like to think that Zoey could sense that Luca needed a bit of love, just like how she needed a bit of love after Benny. Zoey did not give up on life after Benny died and is now a happy and loving dog again. Zoey has shown me the importance of never giving up, even during unfortunate situations, and that you always need someone with whom you can relate especially during tough times.

When we got Luca, I felt as if he could never replace Benny. He can't, but I see a lot of Benny in Luca. Luca loves to lick everyone and everything he sees, just like Benny. He loves to play with Zoey, and he is just as bossy and sassy as Benny used to be.

I've also learned a lot about perseverance through my many years as a drummer and percussionist. Do you remember the old TV show Hawaii 5-0? Well, I certainly do. Let me tell you why. It was the summer of 2021, and I was playing the drums at music camp for the theme song of Hawaii 5-0. I just couldn't get it right. It was the day before the concert and our instructor, Miss Janine, stopped the band mid-song, looked directly at me and simply stated: "Jacob, you aren't playing it right. We're going to run it one more time and if you can't get it down, we're going to have to cut it. I know you can do better than this."

I closed my eyes, took a deep breath, and started to count off the band. While playing, I knew that if I messed up even a single beat that would mean that all the hard work by everyone over the past few weeks of camp would all be in vain. So, I kept playing, trying not to overthink the song and I just played what I knew. When the song ended, Miss Janine came up to me and said, "We're gonna keep it in."

In retrospect, I realize that Miss Janine holding me to such a high standard helped me develop not just into the musician I am now, but into a person who is willing to do the hard work and persevere to achieve excellence.

Miss Janine taught me that in music, as in life, every note counts, and you won't get there if you give up.

FORGIVENESS

One thing my family has taught me is that relationships with friends and family are essential to living a meaningful life and that during a relationship that spans decades, people will inevitably do or say things that are hurtful. This is why kindness toward other people and the ability to forgive are essential to maintaining long-term relationships. As my Great-Grandma Emma used to say, "When you hold onto resentment, you are holding a person prisoner and that person is you." This demonstrates how being a kind and compassionate person is beneficial to both the person giving and receiving kindness.

An essential part of being a kind person is the capacity to forgive another person. Forgiveness is acknowledging that others can make mistakes and valuing the relationship enough to accept an apology and being able to move on and not hold the mistake against the other person. Many times, my dogs have done the wrong thing, from going to the bathroom in the house or tearing up furniture. To have a good relationship with your dog, you have to learn to forgive them for their mistakes. It is still okay to train them to change their behavior, but simply getting mad at them does not help at all. Of course, this is a lesson that should be applied to humans as well as canines!

Benny loved to watch TV with my dad, even if he could not understand what was happening on the TV. He always made sure to keep his face looking at the TV, as if he wanted to let my dad know he cared about what he was watching. After Benny got sick and eventually passed away, I felt incredibly sad as a part of my childhood had vanished. Eventually, I have come to terms with the passing of Benny. However, I still miss him every day. I remember getting woken up early in the morning by my dad and being told Benny had passed away. I remember seeing his emotionless face at the vet and having to say goodbye to Benny for the last time. When Benny died, I realized how grateful I was that I had forgiven him for the mistakes he made while he was alive. I didn't carry any negative feelings towards him and that made his passing so much easier to handle. I could only imagine what it must be like to have a loved one pass and be still carrying unforgiven feelings towards that person. I realize how important it is for me to forgive my friends and relatives for any mistakes they have made. I also realize how important it is to forgive myself for mistakes I've made. Forgiveness is important towards others and towards oneself.

PATIENCE

Patience is waiting and being calm and tolerant during an event you do not like. My first dog, Benny, began his life in a home where the family did not care for him nor treat him well. He was turned over to a rescue shelter and had to wait and watch as other dogs were adopted over him. He had to be patient and wait for a family to bring him home. Another example of patience is how Benny would often take a long time to go to the bathroom because of his medical issues and because he liked to take his time. This meant that whoever was walking him would have to patiently wait for him to go.

Every day, multiple times a day, I walk our dogs. This task isn't always fun, as all of my dogs love to take their sweet time going to the bathroom. Sometimes, it can take ten to twenty minutes for them to finally do their business. Sometimes, they decide they don't need to go at that moment and refuse to go at all. In that case, I take them out again until they eventually decide to go. This daily routine of walking our dogs has taught me how to be patient, even during times when I really want to rush things. I have to be both attentive and patient when walking the dogs. We live in a part of the country where there are tons of wild animals such as coyotes, mountain lions, snakes, and all sorts of dangerous animals could potentially attack our dogs if I am not careful. Along with learning patience, I have been learning to pay attention to small and seemingly unimportant details as I have to do so in order to ensure our dogs stay safe during walks. I also have to be attentive to them to make sure they don't eat or get access to objects they think are food. If that happens, I have to make sure to remove the objects from their mouths. I also must make sure they have no ticks or other bugs on them which happens in our community. It takes a lot of patience to work with the dogs and make sure that they remain safe, healthy, and happy.

Healthy Lifestyle

Exercise is performing physical or mental activities to improve health. Walking dogs is great exercise for us and the dog. I used to walk one of our dogs, Benny, all throughout my neighborhood which tired him out for a bit. This kept him in great shape and also helped me get an easy twenty to thirty minutes of extra exercise every day. This exercise can also be a fun way to spend time when you are bored. Running around with your dog gives them exercise but also provides you with exercise. Having a dog really helps keep people in shape.

Sometimes, the dogs enjoy a good walk in the park. They can meet new people and other dogs so it's a type of social exercise as well. Along with that, I can meet new people during these walks in the park. I can meet all different kinds of people because dogs can give me a great excuse to go outside and engage in public life. I meet older people, younger people, or really any age group or type of person.

We would sometimes take our dogs to a specific park that they loved. They walked around the park as if they owned it even though we lived a good distance away from the park. We would put both dogs into a wagon but only Benny would stay in the wagon as Zoey liked to explore on her own.

Benny used to love to "chase" lizards as his way of chasing them to ensure they did not invade our house. He would sit by a window or door and bark at the lizards until they ran away. Even when they seemed to not hear Benny, he made sure he barked repeatedly for hours at a time. He would surely drive fear into all the lizards in our neighborhood. After his death, the lizards must have felt as if they could finally roam our backyard safely once again.

Sleep is very important for humans and dogs. Dogs have tons of energy and need constant attention so getting to sleep whenever you can is vital to raising a dog. If you stay up late into the night, you won't be able to give enough attention to your dog which can cause your dog to get into trouble if you are distracted. Getting a good night's sleep is very important for not just your dog, but also for you. Our dogs love to sleep all the time. Somehow, their daily schedule of eating, drinking, and walking tires them out a ton. They spend hours at a time sleeping to recover their energy. Sometimes, they decide to sleep with me in my room, which helps me sleep as it is comforting to know my dogs like to be with me.

A healthy lifestyle also pertains to playing an instrument like I do with the drums. When people think about music and which instruments are the hardest or easiest, they will oftentimes mention the drums as one of the easier instruments to learn and practice. However, they could not be more wrong about that. Playing the drum set requires a different breed of musician; someone who has a brain that can play multiple pieces of music at the same time, consistently.

I remember one time at music camp, which I attended ever since I began playing music in the 4th grade, and being allowed to sit down on this certain drum set stool. The set was encased in this massive array of percussion which I had little to no clue how to use effectively. Playing that kit, I began to understand the drums better and how to separate the functioning of my arms and legs from each other, at least in my brain. I could eventually play different beats with different limbs, which is much harder than it sounds. It is incredibly natural for every limb to play the same thing and hit everything at the same time, but for music like the drums, that just won't suffice. You would need to be able to play 8th notes on the hi-hat, half notes on the snare and bass, and be able to fill on all the instruments. This would be considered a fairly basic and easy rhythm to play. To play more complex drumbeats, your brain will be put through the process of having to concentrate on not succumbing to the urge to play the same thing on multiple drums. If this were to happen unintentionally, it can really mess up the groove. You will have to be able to repeat the incredibly complex groove over and over again throughout the song, all at an incredibly precise tempo (speed). Sometimes, that tempo will change, the drum beat you are playing may change, or your drumbeat will be interrupted by a drum fill, and then you will have to instantly go back into the drumbeat, without missing a beat, literally. And if at any time during this, you slow down or speed up even a tiny bit, it can very easily throw off the entire band as they mainly rely on you, the drummer, to keep a steady tempo and stay in time with everyone else. My point in telling you all this is that drumming is an actually physical and mental exercise. It's a part of a healthy lifestyle. Being a drummer is actually very similar to being an athlete. If anyone ever tries to tell you how easy the drum set is to play, just know that drums are one of the most difficult, complex, and challenging instruments to play.

VALUES INTO ACTION

It is very easy to say you believe in something. However, it's your actions that truly matter. You need to show that you care, not just say that you care.

I take great pride in my videography skills, particularly because I have the privilege of using my skills to showcase the accomplishments of my peers. I have been responsible for travelling with my high school sports teams, recording videos for their teams, and helping with other projects as well. These tasks could be as simple as interviewing athletes, coaches, and administrators or as complex as editing videos and recording and analyzing the statistics of the players. These tasks can get complicated as I have to balance my role as a leader of the videography department at my school with the fact that I was on many of my school's sports teams. For example, I played on the school's varsity flag football team, the varsity soccer team, of which I was a captain, and the varsity baseball team where I was the starting 2nd baseman. I had to balance the tasks of performing to the best of my abilities on the field, ensuring that I gave the best chance for my teams to win, while also focusing on recording the sports teams. I had to be available to travel with any sports team that needed to be filmed, while also being available to play and practice for my own teams. After I recorded the games for the sports teams, I edited all of the long footage down into bite sized highlight reels, making sure to include all the important events that happened in each game, while also keeping the videos from being too long. I also keep track of the stats of each game and make sure to share them with each of the teams, for them to improve their performance for the next game and beyond. I take great pride in my work at my school as it is presented in front of the entire school every week, so I always want to bring forth my best work.

To do so, I made sure to collaborate with the rest of the members of the videography department at my school. Asking for input from the other videography members allows me to put forth my best work. I have also done videography for music, school events, school plays, and much more. Filming, editing, and sharing these events has opened my eyes to all the unique and diverse groups of people that are at my school. I can share the things that people at my school enjoy doing with the rest of the school. I love to make sure everyone's voices and hobbies are able to be showcased and that no one feels as if they are being ignored. That is the beauty of videography and broadcasting; you can showcase what people love doing, allowing people to discover new things they may have never found out about otherwise.

I didn't start off playing on the drum set. For many years, I had to stick with just playing one instrument at a time, and that was fun. But as I grew older, I became increasingly interested in playing in a "big band" type of environment. When I saw my first drum set, it was like meeting a new puppy, which I have experienced twice so far. I fell in love with playing on a drum set. It just felt natural and at home banging away and playing the music that I had previously heard coming from my phone. For years now, I have loved to just turn on music on my phone and try to play the music. I have played hundreds of songs with other musicians, which is a feeling unlike anything else. When everyone is playing their parts to the best of their ability, you just get absorbed into the music. It is a sort of meditative experience in some ways. It feels amazing and I wouldn't trade it for anything.

At school, I played the drums in the school band. Every day, while sludging through the, at times, boring school day, I was always anticipating my band class. Whether it be me playing the bells, the timpani, or sometimes when I was lucky enough to play the drum set for a song, I loved playing in my school band. I played my heart out and improved my musical skills every day. Near the end of the year, we would host a musical performance at a nearby high school. This event was what everyone looked forward to every year and we always did our best when the time came around. I remember being incredibly nervous every single time I went to play in these performances. After I got on the stage, I felt calm, and my nerves subsided. We always had to wait for the younger musicians to finish their songs, but when my group got on the stage, I felt a peace come over me. Hundreds of people were watching me on the stage, so I do admit I wasn't completely free of my nerves, but the feeling of the crowd cheering was unlike anything else.

Whenever I am playing my drums, I am truly at peace. I can relax, unlike during the mundane activities of most of the day. Sitting down at the drum stool in the band room at my school, I pick up my sticks and start banging away on the kit. Whether it be rock and roll, jazz, funk, or whatever genre, I love just simply spending hours at a time, playing the drums and not worrying about school or life outside of music.

Drums have taught me so much about life. For example, before I picked up the drumsticks, I struggled to stay still. However, after years of playing the drums during band class, I have learnt how to control my attention to the point where it is no longer an issue for me. Along with that, music has immensely improved my confidence. Before I started playing the drums, I was incredibly shy and struggled to talk to anyone that I did not know well. It was difficult to talk to a cashier to order food or to talk on the phone with strangers. I was afraid to go outside my comfort zone.

However, after I started playing the drums, and after I participated and played in a few concerts, my confidence began to slowly but surely build until I could eventually speak to strangers with ease. Looking back on it now, this is how I learned to put values into action. It feels weird how afraid I was of speaking in public, as I have no problem doing it now. I guess I was just extremely self-conscious of how others would think of me when I talked to them. Music has shown me to stay focused on what I can control and try to let go of the rest. I focus on understanding my values and then finding ways to put these values into action.

We all make mistakes whether it's during a concert or with a family member, and it's important that we accept ourselves and others for being human and not being perfect. I've learned to focus on doing the best I can and being kind to others, especially when they make a mistake. In music, most mistakes aren't even noticed by the audience. That understanding helped me to relax and enjoy myself a lot more. Knowing this, allows us to face our fears in a much more effective way. Playing music and all of life becomes much more enjoyable when you can relax with this understanding. I have never had more enjoyable experiences than the nights when our band played the music that we had practiced for months putting our hard work into action and feeling the results of our work. This work is not always fun, but it's certainly rewarding in so many ways. For months, we practice and fail, until eventually, for ten to fifteen minutes, we must put all our fears aside and play what we know with every bit of heart we can muster. When we finish, the feeling of performing to the best of your abilities is unlike anything else.

HOBBIES

One lesson I've learned is that it is important to have activities and interests about which you are passionate. Hobbies are vitally important. Too many kids in my generation fill their free time with electronics, scrolling social media, or basically just zoning out on digital junk food. It can be addictive to use electronics to fill your free time. I actually think those products are designed to be addictive to increase usage and profits for that industry! I think it takes a conscious effort to turn away from mindlessly consuming electronics and focus your free time on a non-digital hobby. For me, the rewards of having non-digital hobbies far outweigh the challenge of making them a priority.

If you can find hobbies, your enjoyment of life will skyrocket. My favorite hobbies are playing drums, exercising, and spending time with my dogs. If you could count sleep as a hobby that would definitely be on the list!

One of my longest running and favorite hobbies is playing the drums. Whether it be playing in a formal wind ensemble alongside a group of other percussionists, practicing alone in my garage, or playing in a small band. I love everything about playing the drums. So let me tell you the story of how I came to play and love the drums. I have been enthralled by the act of simply hitting the snare, the toms, and the cymbals ever since I was a young kid in 4th grade. It started when my friends encouraged me to join the new band class. I was reluctant to join at first, but when I got there, it all seemed to click. It was as if I were born to play the drums; It just felt natural to do so. Whether it was playing the drum set or playing the snare drum, it all just felt natural, and it brought me peace. Do you have a hobby that brings you peace? I am so blessed to have found the drums. If you don't have a hobby that brings you peace, keep looking. No matter what has changed in my life, drums remained a constant activity inside and outside of school. As I grew up, I continued playing the drums. I played in concerts with my school, took lessons, and got more and more into the deeper intricacies of music that I may have never learned if I hadn't picked up the drums. I have played more genres than I could even name, and I have met so many new types of people through playing the drums. I hope to never quit playing music. It's become a core part of who I am.

After training on a small drum pad at home, my parents decided to get me my own drum set. It was an electric drum set because my sisters would never forgive my parents if they had gotten me a real drum set with all the noise that it involves. I spent my free time banging away and having a blast. Every day after school, I got home and instantly sat down on my drum set, turned on music, and started playing for hours. I took lessons online which were so convenient and helpful with my development. I had a bell kit right next to my drum set which I used to practice songs. I spent hours and hours working on my skills. The drum set was right across from my bed which allowed me to start playing music whenever I wanted, no matter the time and no matter the situation. All I had to do was plug in my headphones to the drum set and start banging away.

This drum set was an amazing addition to my life as it allowed me to practice at home, when before I used to have to wait until I got to school to practice. I could also customize the sounds that came out of the drum set, and I could also connect my drum set to my headphones, so I didn't disturb the rest of my family. Whenever I was assigned new music for school, all I had to do was go home and go to my room and I would be able to easily practice my music.

The bell kit is the stereotypical small piano like instrument that you hit with two small mallets. I preferred to be playing on the drum set compared to the bell kit, but I was required to also play on the bell kit. Whether it be playing on my bell kit or playing whatever song that comes to mind on my drum set, I love playing drums at my house. Whenever I play the drums, I forget about anything that is bothering me and just jam away either by myself or with my friends.

Another hobby that adds to the quality of my life is exercising. Studies have shown that exercising greatly boosts not just your physical health but also your mental health. Whenever I exercise, I feel incredibly happy and rejuvenated. Not only do I get into better shape while exercising, I also simply become happier and less stressed for the rest of the day and beyond. Even on days I don't feel like exercising, I'm always glad I did it once I'm done.

The other thing I've noticed is that the more often I exercise, the more I actually look forward to it. During the school year, my involvement with three varsity sports teams ensures that I get enough exercise! During the summer and school breaks, I've gotten into the habit of working out right after I wake up. At first, I hated waking up earlier than I "needed" to but, after a couple of weeks, working out first thing became a part of my daily routine. Just like brushing your teeth in the morning, it's usually best to just do exercise and not think too much about it. This summer, I started working out in the morning. I ended up with more mental and physical energy. This is just one way you can prioritize a hobby that enhances your life.

One other hobby that I want to share is playing with our dogs (I have so many more hobbies that I enjoy but I don't need to share every one of them with you!). Dogs, and pets in general, have a way of boosting your happiness and mental health by just being unconditionally adorable and kind to you. No matter how difficult the day way, dogs are always there to love you. Whether it be going on a run with the dogs, taking them to the park, or throwing them toys in the house, I always love playing with our dogs. The more time I spend with my dogs, the happier I am.

Having hobbies in your life is vital to staying happy and enjoying life. Without hobbies, life usually boils down to sleeping, eating, and working. That's not a recipe for a happy, peaceful, and productive life. When I spend more time on the activities that enhance life and less time on a plugged-in device, I am happier and feel more in control of my life.

FAMILY

L ove is caring for someone without conditions and that is what a family and community is all about. I have learned a lot about the importance of family, whether it be the family into which I was born, or the community I experienced at Camp Kesem, through music, and through playing sports.

I mentioned Camp Kesem earlier in the book and now I'll let you know a bit about this wonderful camp and charity. Camp Kesem is a free, sleepaway camp for kids affected by one or more of their parents having cancer. My mom has breast cancer, and we are so lucky that she's doing well and still here with us. When my mom was going through treatment for her breast cancer, she discovered Camp Kesem and she and my dad decided that my three sisters and I would spend the summer at the UCLA Camp Kesem. I turned seven right before my first year at camp and I was nervous I would get homesick being away from my parents. My sisters were worried that camp would be all about talking about cancer and not much fun. Kesem is a regular summer camp full of sports, music, and all the other fun stuff most camps have. It also is a caring place where all the campers are experiencing the same awful situation of having a parent with cancer. Thus, part of each day involves having a chance to talk about some very difficult feelings that each of us has experienced. If we want to, we can share with the group or individually with the counsellors. It's a truly healing and nurturing place.

Camp Kesem is all about having a ton of fun while surrounded by peers and counselors who just understand what it's like to have a parent with cancer. Even at the age of seven, I had so much fun and felt so much support that I barely had time to be homesick!

One of the most powerful lessons I learned about at Camp Kesem is the importance of family. I remember sitting in the audience at a camp wide event called "Empowerment" where everyone had the opportunity to stand up in front of the camp and share their experience with having a parent with cancer: I remember wanting to go up and share my story about how my mom got cancer and the effects it had on my family. I asked my sisters to go up with me, but they were all too scared to share in public, so I gathered my courage, and I went up in front of the camp on my own. Not long into trying to share my story, I started to break down crying and I could not find the strength to speak any more. To my surprise, my sisters came up to me to support me and one of my sisters took over telling our story as she knew I wasn't able to finish. I'll never forget that moment and the way my sisters demonstrated their support and love for me by showing me how the power of family and their love for me, their little brother, overcame their fear of public speaking.

I'll tell you more about Camp Kesem later in the book, but I want to mention a little more about our dogs and how they have taught me a lot about the importance of family. Before my family had a dog, my father, like so many other dads, was adamant that he did not want a dog. He was worried he and my mom would end up doing all the work involved in taking care of a dog and that my siblings and I would quickly lose interest. However, after we adopted our first dog Benny, my dad loved him more than anyone on the planet. He would fall asleep on the couch with Benny by his side and he would talk in a baby voice with Benny, something very out of character for him to do. Getting a dog can shift someone's entire mindset and turn them into someone who loves dogs more than anything else.

And part of being in a family is loving one another even when they aren't at their best. One day while I was at my soccer practice, Benny came to watch and was being petted by the younger sister of one of my teammates. Benny decided it was the right time to pee, so he peed directly on her foot. We had just adopted Benny, and he was not fully potty trained as his original owners didn't think it was important. For a long time, my teammates gave me a hard time about what Benny did, but that did not change how much I loved him as he was a member of my family. In a family, you support each other and forgive when we make mistakes.

I have heard horror stories of people hitting their dogs if they pee or poop in places where they are not supposed to go. I could never imagine ever doing this to one of our dogs, no matter what they did. It horrifies me that anyone could ever do that to a dog. After we had Benny for a few years, he got better at waiting to go to the bathroom (and sometimes even told us when he needed to go!). We were able to help him potty train by simply rewarding him when he did what we wanted him to do.

We found out from the shelter where we adopted Benny that his prior family hadn't treated him well. Benny would always be afraid of older men with walking canes, so our theory was that an older man must have treated him badly. Thinking about this even now breaks my heart. Knowing Benny's history helped us better understand and correct some of his behavior. And part of being a family is seeking to understand and help one another.

Benny would always have to wear a diaper at night as he never truly had the ability to hold in his pee, especially as he got older and sicker. He went from the energetic and vibrant dog we saw when we first got him, to a slow and sickly dog near the time of his death. However, we always loved him the same. Even when we had to leave him at an emergency veterinary clinic for a few days so they could keep him in an oxygen chamber box because he was very sick with pneumonia, we visited him every day as we would have for any family member. We loved Benny so much.

No matter how sick Benny got and no matter how close we all knew he was to death, everyone in our family loved him and knew the best way to help him was to be incredibly loving and caring to not just him, but also to each other. Dogs can sense when people around them are angry at each other and we all know that it would not be good for his health if he was constantly sad about that. That inspired us to be nicer to each other.

When Benny first saw Zoey, he probably just thought she was another dog he saw on a walk. Little did he know he would spend the rest of his life being pestered and annoyed by his adorable little sister. At first, he really seemed to be annoyed with her. She would always try to jump on him to play, to which he did not take kindly. Benny was already getting older when we got Zoey, and Zoey was a very active and outgoing puppy, so she didn't understand that Benny did not want to play. However, as the years went on, Benny started to like Zoey more and more. He began to play with her. She still annoyed him plenty, but Benny began to truly love her.

Benny always cared about everyone in our family. For a twenty-pound dog, he acted and behaved as if he were one hundred and fifty pounds. His bark sounded as if he were at least ten times his actual size. He commanded respect from everyone even if he didn't fit the stature of a guard dog. However, he would never hurt anyone ever, yet he would always make sure to let us know someone was there if they were not supposed to be there. I miss Benny so much.

COMMUNITY

Usually, when people talk about having a parent with cancer, it is usually in a completely negative sense. However, my mom getting cancer did result in at least a tiny bit of good for my family. Don't get me wrong, I would trade anything for my mom to have never gotten cancer, but life had other plans for us.

When my mom first got cancer, I was distraught. I was still super young, yet I still understood the possible implications involved in a cancer diagnosis. For a while, I felt so lost and afraid that my mom might get very sick. As I mentioned in the last section, Camp Kesem truly made such a big difference in my life. I have gone to the camp almost every year for more than a decade ever since.

Camp Kesem is a free sleepaway summer camp for kids whose parents have experienced cancer and sadly there are tons of kids in this situation. It might be cliché to say this, but Kesem truly is my home away from home. Camp Kesem provides a way for me to talk with people who have experienced things that many other people could never understand. I'm so grateful my mom found a way for all four of us to have fun at a summer camp while also being able to share our story with people who truly understand. The kindness and compassion we experienced at Camp Kesem was transformative for all four of us.

Even though I was just seven years old the first time I went to Camp Kesem, I still remember every detail of that first summer. Drop off for Camp Kesem begins at a park where kids get to meet their counselors and fellow campers, say goodbye to parents, and then board the bus to the camp site. Going to camp was the first time I had ever been away from my parents for more than one night and I was pretty nervous. Fortunately, I was comforted because my three big sisters were there with me.

After a very long bus ride spent staring at the mountain scenery, my sisters and I finally arrived at the campsite along with dozens of other campers and counselors. We got off the bus and after a short wait, my camp group and I took our luggage to our cabin. After this, we spent the remainder of the day getting introduced to the other people at the camp and playing a few games. After doing this and eating dinner, it was time for bed. It took me a while to finally fall asleep as I was incredibly homesick, but eventually my eyelids closed, and I drifted off to sleep.

The next morning, I was woken up by counselors cheerfully barging into our bunk, loudly singing songs to wake us up. I tried to stay in my bed for as long as possible, but eventually I had to get up for the day. That day, my group went on a zip line which was a great time. As the hours went by, I started to enjoy being at the camp and almost forgot about my life outside of camp. After the zip line, we went swimming and I loved it. I went down a water slide over and over again which was a blast.

After lunch, my group did arts and crafts, making whatever we wanted. During this, I got to meet new people and made a bunch of new friends. I don't remember everything else that happened during that first day, but I do remember that I had a great time. During dinner, my group and I talked and made jokes for a while and eventually the camp came together and sang a song to close out the day. Our cabin then came together and talked about our day and the good and bad that happened. After this, my friends and I forced our counselors to tell us a bedtime story.

The next morning, it was more of the same. Getting woken up by loud music and singing, going to breakfast, and then regrouping. On this day, my group and I went swimming again and it was fun. Slowly my stress and anxiety were lifting feeling all the love and support around me. It was hot that summer, but I remember the cool temperature of the lake water. After the swim, my group and I went and played some ping pong and other games in the game room. After this, my group and I went upstairs and sang karaoke and sang a bunch of great songs. After this, we had a rest hour where I read a book. It was a real book and not a digital book.

I was very happy when the hour ended, and we were able to get back to hanging out as a group doing whatever. Next up was archery, which isn't a skill of mine, but I still had a blast. I completely missed the target almost every time, yet I strangely really enjoyed it. When I wasn't shooting my arrows into the dirt, I spent most of archery talking with the other campers. I don't remember what we were talking about, but that does not really matter. I remember being happy.

After this, we went to a tree house and played ice breaker games. I remember this tree house having a very small zip line that everyone would use. After the tree house, I do not really remember what happened next until after dinner, when the group and I were told that our unit was called the green unit. They had us walk around blindfolded for a minute and then made us drink sprite from a bowl. Then they made us eat sour candy, telling us it was a bug. Thinking about it right now as I am writing, I find it funny how my 7-year-old self was terrified during this. We went to dinner and then I went to sleep so tired from all the activities.

The next morning, we went on the zip line again, which was fun again. We then played capture the flag and then we played soccer, which I loved as I played club soccer around this time. After this, we went to the pool and played "wipeout". A bunch of floaties were put into the pool and we had to race across the pool as fast as possible. I was not the best at this, but I did love spraying the other racers with water as they ran across the course. After this, we participated in an event called "messy activities". By the name alone, you can guess what happened during this. A bunch of shaving cream, paint, and other messy stuff was shot around and everyone got extremely messy. After cleaning ourselves up in the shower, most of the camp went on a long hike to a giant rock a few miles from the campsite. We also sang songs along the way. After we finally arrived at the big rock, we climbed up on it and took a group photo of the entire camp. To close out this day, there was a movie watching event where we watched The Sandlot. I remember not knowing or caring about baseball until watching this movie. After watching the movie, I fell in love with baseball. It was an amazing movie, and I am thankful I got introduced to baseball by this movie. After the movie, I showered, and we went to dinner once again.

To start off the next day, my group and I went on a long hike around the camp, looking at the mountain views and just talking with each other. After this, there was a special event called "Empowerment" where anyone could talk about their story and experience with cancer. It was a very sad, but important part of the week. There was a lot of crying every time someone shared their story of cancer destroying a happy family. Even though it is very hard to listen to the heart-wrenching stories, it is inspiring to see people opening up about their experience and being vulnerable.

I remember wanting to go up and share my story about how my mom got cancer and the effects it had on me and my family. I asked my sisters to go up with me, but they were all too scared of public speaking to go up, and so was I to an extent. So, I went on my own and started to tell our story. As I mentioned, I started to break down crying. I think this was the first time I cried about mom and her cancer. I could not find the strength to speak anymore. Quickly, to my surprise, my sisters came up to me to support me and one of my sisters took my place in telling our story as she knew I wouldn't be able to finish it. I will never forget the love my sisters showed me in that moment.

Later that day, there was a giant carnival for the camp. There was a giant inflatable obstacle course, a cotton candy and flavored ice station, and so much more. I remember seeing all these kids being so happy despite having such a painful situation at home. I remember thinking how kind all the counsellors were to us.

I remember my friends and I would play a game they called "gaga ball" during the carnival. Gaga ball was a game where you hit the ball with your hands and try to get the ball to hit the feet of other people to eliminate them from the game. Thus, basically the opposite of soccer. At the time, I was very little and thus not very good at gaga ball compared to the other people playing against me, who were way older than me. Only after growing up and getting bigger have I eventually gotten good at gaga ball.

During the carnival, there was also swimming, which I personally did not participate in as I preferred getting cotton candy, playing gaga ball, and racing my friends on the obstacle course. After the carnival, there was a talent show, where I performed. Along with a counselor, we did a performance where I jumped and flipped off the counselor repeatedly, which I found very fun and impressive at the time. I don't know if it looked the same to the audience, but I would like to believe it did.

I remember feeling so tired at that point and wanting to just go to sleep. However, I stayed awake, barely, and watched the remainder of the talent show. After this, we sang more songs and then we talked for a while in our cabin about our week. After this, a bunch of my friends talked about random stuff for a while until we eventually got too tired and fell asleep for one more time. When we woke up, it was time to pack all our stuff, go to breakfast, talk to each other about the entire week, and start to say our goodbyes.

After breakfast, we watched a long video of pictures taken of us all week. I liked watching the video as it was basically a giant recap of an incredibly adventurous week. After the video, we loaded onto the bus and began the long bus ride back to the park. On this bus ride, one of my counselors let me play video games on his iPhone, which I loved so much. Along with that, a bunch of people played guessing games and other time wasters. When we got back to the park, we unpacked our luggage from the bus. I remember getting off the bus and looking for my family, and seeing both of my parents, along with our dog, Benny. They were waiting for us.

We brought our luggage to the car before returning to the park to do a group-based award ceremony. I don't remember which award I won, but I do remember winning one. After saying goodbye to my friends, and after asking the counselors for their name tags, my family and I left to go back home. We talked about the camp activities for the entire drive home. Cancer was the last thing on my mind.

The next summer, I was incredibly excited to return to camp. Packing my stuff for camp, I was happy to go off to camp which was a vast difference compared to the previous summer. The year before, I was scared to leave home and have to talk about having a mom with a life-threatening illness. In contrast, this time I felt completely fine, very much looking forward to it. Driving to the park to get dropped off, I listened to music on my iPod touch.

When we got dropped off, I actually wanted my parents to leave because I was so excited about camp; not because I didn't love them, but because I was excited to see my friends. This was truly my new home away from home.

I met up with my friends from last year and chatted with them. We talked about what had been happening so far that summer and during the school year. After my parents said their goodbyes and left, we packed all the luggage into the buses, just like last year, and drove off to the same campsite. After we got there, a few of my friends and I went to the tree house to play on the zipline. After a good while of playing around, we got together with the rest of our group and brought out stuff to our cabins, just like the previous year. I happened to be placed in the yellow unit this year, the unit right after the green unit where I had been the prior year. This year, we started off the week by introducing ourselves while sitting together in the tree house.

I remember our group played a game where we had to make a dance move that corresponded to our camp names that we created for ourselves. At Camp Kesem, every camper and counselor are required to create a camp name to be used in place of their real name. The idea is that camp should represent a place where you can leave your regular life issues behind. My first year, I was called "Spike", but this year I was called "Avenger".

After we finished with this icebreaker, we went to dinner. During this dinner, there was an eating competition for three counselors. They had to eat some disgusting assortment of condiments and whatever else the kitchen staff had available. It was truly disgusting to watch, but incredibly funny at the same time. I do not want to imagine how ill each person must have felt later that night.

After the usual singing to close out the night, and the cabin chat as well, we all went to bed. The next morning, we went to breakfast and then went on a short hike. During this hike, a guy dressed up in a costume that looked like bigfoot ran out of the forest and all the campers and I chased him down. Of course, it turned out to be just a counselor. After the hike, we all went back to the campsite and had a rest hour. We played a card game called "Exploding Kittens". I don't remember everything about this card game, but it had something to do with pandas and unicorns. After the hour was complete, we all went to lunch to eat some food and talk some more. After we had finished eating lunch, we went to swim in the pool. On this day, we played the game Sharks and Minnows. I wasn't the best swimmer as I was still very young, so I did not fare well in sharks and minnows. Despite this, I still had a fun time as again, like for most things at Camp Kesem, it is the experience of just hanging out with your friends that makes everything feel special.

Along with playing sharks and minnows, we also played "chicken fight" where one person got on top of another person's shoulders and tried to knock over another person who was doing the same thing. Usually, it was a camper on the shoulders of a counselor as most of us were very young and in turn also very small. I was surprisingly good at knocking the other duo over as I was very strong even for my size. After getting out of the pool and drying off, we went across the camp site and played dodge ball. I loved playing dodge ball as I have always been a very competitive person. Even if I was very, very bad at throwing the ball and catching the ball, I always had an amazing time playing. After a few rounds of dodgeball, we went over to another part of the camp site to tie dye a bunch of white shirts which we would be able to take home after camp ended. I decided to go with the colors red, blue, and orange as I thought that would look the best.

After finishing with the tie dye, we played a bunch of camp games together with a few other groups and also played some basketball, which I was not very good at as I am not very tall. Despite this, I really enjoyed playing sports and talking to each other, even if I did not make a single shot for the entire time we were playing basketball.

After playing basketball, we went over to a beach volleyball court and played a few games of volleyball. I was decent at setting the ball, but similar to how I was too short to do much at basketball, the same could be said for volleyball. Despite this, I tried my best and had a great time. While people were playing volleyball, a bunch of people were playing gaga ball, which I quickly switched over to as I was much better at gaga ball than at volleyball. Over the last year, I improved at gaga ball and could hold my own against the bigger kids much better than I could the year before. I don't remember how I improved so much in a year, but I think I just got better with my hand eye coordination and became a little more agile.

After an hour of playing gaga ball and volleyball, we went off to lunch. This would include us "cooking" "meals" for the counselors. This meal would include whatever food and condiments that we could access. I remember that we made a meal that included hot sauce, water, mustard, sardines, salt, and a ton of even more disgusting ingredients that my mind likely filtered out, so I didn't have to think about it. After serving the "food" to the counselors, we returned to our cabin for the night.

Each of these activities seems minor and insignificant as I write about them, but there is something different at Camp Kesem. There was so much love and compassion there and it was amazing to see so many kids smiling for the first time in a long time. That's what community is all about; lifting each other up.

COLLABORATION

Benny, our oldest dog, used to love to get pampered by anyone who would pamper him. He was basically a person magnet and so we would always meet people when we walked Benny at the park. Benny got as much attention as he could ever want. This trait didn't stop with the next two rescue dogs that we adopted.

Benny was also creative and unique dog who didn't limit himself to activities commonly attributed to canines. On many occasions, Benny would escape out of the front door, and he would run and scramble away to our next-door neighbor's house, where another dog lived. He would scratch at their front door and sit down patiently because he wanted to play with their dog. My sisters always thought he had a crush on the female dog named who lived there. Sadly for Benny, their dog was grumpy and always rejected him. Still, Benny persisted. Whenever he managed to escape from our house, we always knew where to find him!

Benny was the type of dog who always wanted to find friends and collaborate with them to have as much fun as possible. Collaboration is working with a group of people to achieve a common goal. This skill is essential to success in just about every area of life. I've tried to follow Benny's lead and make collaboration a big part of my life whether through videography, sports, or music.

At my school, the best extracurricular activity is Band Club which creates an opportunity for students to form groups with other student musicians who play instruments. I have participated in this club every year I have attended this school as I love to showcase my skills to the school. I also love to create music with other students at my school. Even when I don't get to play the types of music I enjoy, I still love playing the songs. I get to play and listen to new types of music that I would not have heard. I enjoy playing new genres of music and growing my musical skills.

At school, I can practice the drums whenever I have a free period, or before and after school. I love to use the free time I must practice songs for garage band, or songs that I like and that I want to be able to play. Whenever I am there, I get to talk with other musicians who are also practicing, talking about music or just life in general. The band room is a great way to meet new people and build upon the relationships you have made with other people. The band room is also simply a place where people can go to escape the weather. The air-conditioned room allows people to practice music, talk with their friends, and relax from a hard day of schoolwork.

It might not be obvious that videoing events for a future broadcast requires collaboration, but I have found that to be a central requirement of being successful in this endeavor. For this to go well, the people I am videoing and interviewing need to trust me and cooperate with me; to earn that trust I need to demonstrate that I care about them and their sport or event. Ultimately, a sports or fine arts report reflects a collaboration between the videographer and the subjects of the report. That is the beauty of videography and broadcasting; you can showcase what so many people love which enables the viewers to learn about new things which they otherwise would never have discovered.

In addition to being a videographer for my school, I have also played on numerous varsity sports teams at my high school the entire time I have been there. I have played on each of the highest-level teams offered at my school, whether it be flag football, soccer, or baseball. Being captain of the soccer team as well as a consistent starter on all three teams, means that I was given a ton of responsibility to lead by example both on and off the field. As a player, I had to make sure to put forth my best performances every game day while also ensuring that I lifted everyone on my team whenever they needed support. Off the field, I demonstrate my teamwork by getting a peer an icepack after an injury, giving helpful feedback on how to improve their game, or just providing reassurance after something didn't go our way on the field.

Collaboration is demonstrated in different ways in different sports. In baseball, I have roles both on and off the field. On the field, we collaborate on double plays or throwing a player out at second base on a stolen base attempt. Off the field, I work as student manager, meaning I collaborate on off the field matters such as scheduling or reviewing statistics.

While doing behind the scenes work, I also have my on-field responsibilities meaning I need to be at the top of my game with hitting and fielding. On the football team, every aspect of my involvement on the team requires teamwork.

One aspect of how I go above and beyond is that, in addition to being a player on the football team, I am also team manager for the team. In this role, I make sure that all needed athletic supplies are available and ready for each practice or game. On the field, I play on the offensive line, a role that does not usually get a lot of attention when doing the job correctly. The O-line works as a unit to protect our quarterback and give our team the best opportunity to score. Happily, my fellow offensive line teammates exhibit our own collaboration by communicating with each other. I really love the feeling of seeing a fellow teammate make a great play as I know that I helped them through my work on the field. In addition, as one of the senior members on each of my sports teams, I must be a good role model for the younger members of the team and to make sure they give forth their best effort and best sportsmanship. My coaches expect leaders on the team to provide appropriate on-field coaching and constructive criticism and that is a responsibility which I take seriously. My coaches know that I am someone they can rely on to get a task done on and off the field, as I have showcased this ability throughout my time in high school. If they want a drill to be run while they are busy with other work, they often come to me to help lead the drill as they know I am responsible to lead the group. My coaches also know I am someone with whom they can share information about future games and future strategies as I have proven to be a reliable leader. They often ask me for input, as I have consistently demonstrated my extensive knowledge of sports strategy and the ability to apply statistical analysis.

Our dogs have also taught me a lot about collaboration. Everyone in the family needs to chip in and help feed, walk, and play with the dogs. It can't be one person doing all the work regarding the dogs. Every single person needs to help in their own way. This can be via walking the dogs to give them exercise, bringing out food and water for them to eat and drink, or even training them to behave better. If everyone in the family is working together on this common goal of raising a dog, everything becomes much simpler and easier. Working together to raise and train your dogs helped to bring our family closer together and made our relationships stronger. The dogs have brought our family together more than it has ever been. They make us laugh, they cuddle, and they love being with us. It makes every day of life less mundane, and more action packed. Our family would go on many trips with our dogs which we likely never would have gone to without them. These trips were very fun and brought our family closer together while also letting us get outside instead of just sitting inside watching television.

Playing music has also taught me about collaboration. When you focus your ears on the small intricacies of the music that is being played, you can hear a ton of details that you would otherwise never notice and marvel at how the musicians collaborate. For example, in a movie, the type of music and the instrument choice can either build the tension to an extreme point during a scary movie, express the love a character is feeling for another character in a romance movie, or build up an adventurous feeling in an adventure movie. You usually don't think about the musical score while enjoying a movie, but without music, a movie would feel incredibly bland and very boring to watch. Music is an incredibly underrated part of the movie watching experience.

In other forms of media, like video games for example, the same thing can occur. The music being played for a specific level in a video game can make you feel incredibly powerful and can also help create emotions in the viewer just like in a movie. For me, playing an instrument has unlocked a part of my brain that forces me, for the better, to focus on the minor details in music which heavily boosts my enjoyment of the medium. I can notice minor details in other instruments, not just percussion and the drum set. I have learned to be able to hear every little detail in a song to be able to remember where I am in a specific piece, which has allowed me to in turn hear details in songs I hear on the radio. Even though I can now focus more on songs, this hasn't reduced my enjoyment of normal music. I would say it did the opposite. I can now appreciate parts of songs that most people would just completely ignore.

Playing in a big band, a jazz band with a variety of instruments, is an incredible experience to have at one point in your life. When every band member is playing their best and the solos are good, it feels amazing. When I am on the drum set, I am basically the backbone of the group, keeping the rhythm and tempo steady for the rest of the group. A well-timed fill here and there can really improve the vibes of a song. Using the drum set to highlight the parts being played by the other band members can sound really amazing if done correctly. For example, if the trumpet plays a specific part over and over again, sometimes, I could hit my drums to match what they are playing, which heavily boosts the impact of the music.

Simple things like this can really benefit the quality of the song.

In my family, we strive to help each other out as much as possible. For example, if someone needs help with homework, another sibling or a parent will be readily available to go out and help them with whatever questions they may have. This way of life has been heavily boosted by my experience of playing the drums. When I play music with others, there are no winners and losers. Everyone has one common goal and that is creating an amazing piece of music. Unlike in sports like basketball or football, where there are two teams competing against each other, music, for the most part, only includes teammates. I have learned to focus on helping others improve their skills when I am playing with a band, as I know they would do the same, and that the act of people helping each other will only benefit the quality of our work. For example, I often remember situations where a fellow drummer was having a very hard time understanding a part, so I would offer my help to them for the group to improve.

In competitive sports, some teammates won't want to help their own teammates as they could see their teammates as competing for spots on the team. In music, this usually isn't an issue. A musician in a band usually is not concerned about losing a "position" as those positions are usually predetermined beforehand. There really is no reason to refuse to help someone in a musical environment as you really gain nothing by only working on yourself. In fact, you may be harmed in the long run as others won't be open to helping you, whenever you are having trouble with a piece.

Also, for me at least, I enjoy selflessly helping others. It gives me a happy feeling when I know that I have truly helped someone improve themselves. Playing the drums for nearly a decade now, I have realized that working together with others is much more beneficial and enjoyable than working alone. The drum section often has a ton of band members, all playing similar but distinct parts that complement each other and increase the overall quality of a musical piece. If the drum section was fighting with another section, not wanting to allow another person to gain any advantages over anyone, the quality of the work they all produce would be heavily diminished. The quality would be so much better if they collaborated in a positive way.

It may be difficult to help others when you have done so much hard work on your own without help, but those who help others without expecting anything in return are those who will be helped themselves down the line. That's what I have learned from my experience playing the drums. It may sound like a cliché, but good things do indeed happen to good people who help others.

LISTENING

The last lesson that I want to share with you may be the most important one. It is listening. A baseball coach I know once said that we have two ears and one mouth so we should listen twice as much as we talk. That's an important lesson. Listening is an essential element of communication and paying attention to what is happening around you is an important part of that. My dogs have a way to inform the entire family that they need to go to the bathroom. A small bell hangs on the door so that they ring whenever they need to go outside and this allows us to know when our dogs need to go. Listening to what your dog needs is crucial to having a happy and healthy dog. You need to know when your dog isn't feeling well, when they are hungry, and when they want to play. We learn this by listening; by paying attention which means that we stop talking for a period of time and simply listen.

CONCLUSION

If you've gotten this far, I really appreciate you spending the time to read this book. I just have one more thing to share before you close this book and put it away. I hope my book can help you find strategies to cope the next time you face a challenging experience.

The word "STICK-TO-IT-IVENESS" represents my belief that success and happiness in life comes from ensuring that your life choices represent your values and putting those values into action on a consistent basis. I wrote this book with the goal of sharing the lessons I've learned along my journey to help younger kids as they grow up and face similar challenges. I am grateful for the mentorship I have received from a wide variety of people: my parents, sports coaches, music teachers, and many more I cannot even begin to name. I hope that the small resource of my book can help provide guidance through life's difficulties by sharing some of the lessons and coping strategies I've learned along the way.

Don't give up. Stick with it. Practice STICK-TO-IT-IVENESS!!!

Thank you again.

Best,

Jacob

ACKNOWLEDGEMENTS

T hank you, Mom and Dad, for being there for me no matter what. Thank you, Mom, for driving me to every soccer practice and to every school event, even when you were tired. Thank you, Dad, for always watching sports with me, and for taking me to see all your favorite bands. I love spending that time with you, even if I am 40 years younger than everyone else at the concerts.

Thank you, Gramma Cele and Papa Joe, for always being unconditionally loving and supportive, and for teaching me to love chess. Thank you, Miss Janine, for mentoring me and pushing me to be the best musician I could be. Thank you, Mr. Larry, for teaching me how to play the drum set and always helping me learn any song I asked. Thank you to my three sisters for being supportive and kind to me even when I was an annoying little brother and asked so many questions. And most importantly, thank YOU, for reading my book and I hope you enjoyed it.

INFORMATION ABOUT THE AUTHOR

Jacob is a senior at a high school in Southern California. He has played the drums for most of his life and has no plans to stop. His many interests include music, sports, videography, and his two dogs, Zoey and Luca. After college, Jacob plans to pursue a business career, likely in sports or music management. Jacob is the youngest of four children.

www.ingramcontent.com/pod-product-compliance
Lightning Source LLC
Chambersburg PA
CBHW031625040426

42452CB00007B/684